Stop Dieting, Change Your Life and Lose Weight

Lose Big Fat Fast, Forget the Diet and Improve Yourself

Jason Guise

Table of Contents

Conclusion

Introduction

Congratulations on purchasing *Stop Dieting, Change Your Life and Lose Weight,* and thank you for doing so.

When it comes to losing weight or even leading a healthy life, for that matter, there is no end to the amount of advice you will find on the internet. In fact, the magazines keep publishing something about fad diets month after month and portray them as the 'breakthrough' in the weight loss industry. I'm sure every one of you has come across an ad at least once in your life that says 'Lose 30 Pounds by Christmas!' But have you ever thought about it scientifically? If you reduce your daily caloric intake, it's no wonder that you are going to shed pounds but is that process going to be healthy for your body and long-term health? No. So, what should you do instead? That is exactly what you will learn here in this book.

Fad diets are becoming popular in our world almost every day, and do you know why? It's because they are heavily marketed by the corporate giants for their own monetary benefits. As the novelty of one fad diet ad fades away, they start pushing another one to those same heights. But there is a way out of this toxic cycle and that is through engaging in healthy habits that you will learn here.

There are plenty of books on this subject on the market; thanks again for choosing this one! Every effort was made to ensure it is full of as much useful information as possible. Please enjoy!

Chapter 1: Why Dieting is the Biggest Enemy of Weight Loss?

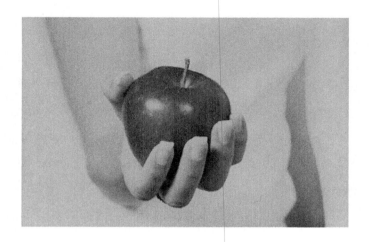

Are you highly concerned about losing extra pounds of weight and so thinking of following a strict diet plan? Well, a lot of individuals like you choose to diet to lose weight. Do you think starving yourself regularly is a good idea for shedding extra pounds? Your response may be yes, but you might be shocked to know that it is certainly not. The truth is that losing weight with the help of dieting has become a worldwide business of multi-million dollars. But no such authentic evidence is available which shows that the result of dieting is people becoming slimmer. Certain evidence does exist, which exhibits an essential fact that the diets related to weight loss programs are not efficient to work properly for the long term. Such diets may also lead to a gain of weight.

Here you will get to know about some of the negative or bad effects of dieting, as well as the necessary information that will help you understand why dieting is treated as the biggest enemy of weight loss.

If you practice dieting in a way that is healthy, it will be beneficial. But, nowadays, a maximum number of people rely on attractive fad diets. Though the fad diets might seem to be appealing as such diets promise to give quick outcomes yet they affect a person's health negatively. Numerous trustworthy studies reveal the fact that instead of losing weight, a maximum number of individuals who follow dieting frequently end up gaining weight over time.

Appetite hormones get multiplied, and that is one major factor behind regaining the lost weight. A person's body increases the production of such hormones that induce hunger when it starts sensing that it lacks muscles and fat. Your body is forced to stay in starvation mode just because of dieting. It can also be dangerous. For example – 'yo-yo' dieting is one of the most popular forms of dieting, which is actually a repeated cycle of gaining, losing, and again gaining the lost weight. This form of dieting affects your health negatively, such as the risk or chance of various heart diseases increases, metabolism slows down, etc.

Usually, diets do not teach people ways of consuming balanced and controlled portions. It does not even allow you to enjoy the food on the whole. It simply teaches or instructs you certain things, such as the foods that need to be restricted and the rapid ways of losing weight. While following the diet, you may lose excessive weight. The actual scenario gets revealed after you stop maintaining your diet. When a person returns to his/her former eating habits and begins to consume a bit more calories, he/she starts gaining weight. This stands to be one of the major reasons why people who run after strict diets usually end up acquiring their lost weight. In a study, around 2,700 people were involved who dieted some time before. Researchers concluded that those people's waist circumferences and body weight were more than those who never followed any sort of diet.

Now, have a look at some other negative effects of dieting that will let you understand why dieting is treated as the biggest enemy of not only your weight loss but also your overall health.

- *Gallstones* – One of the severe side effects of a low-calorie diet is nothing other than gallstones. If a person starts losing weight very rapidly, his/her liver begins secreting excessive cholesterol. This, in turn, may lead to a sufficient quantity of cholesterol inside the bile, which causes gallstones. When an individual suffers from gallstones just because of dieting, he/she may exhibit symptoms like excessive pain in the upper abdomen, vomiting, nausea, indigestion, bloating, severe gas, and heartburn.

- *Lack of various minerals and vitamins* – Dieting means eliminating certain food groups, leading to the deficiency of particular minerals and vitamins. If you consume only one type of food or, say, a handful of a few foods while following a diet and that too for a long period (from a week to a month), your body won't get the other necessary nutrients at all. Restricting the intake of starches like potatoes, rice, bread (whole grain), oatmeal will reduce B vitamins and fiber. When someone cuts out dairy products from his/her diet, it will decrease the main sources of vitamin D, calcium, and protein. If your body does not get the required quantity of calcium, you may be at the risk of getting osteoporosis, broken bones, and stress fractures. If you stop yourself from eating certain fruits, it will lessen certain nutrients, including vitamin A, vitamin C, potassium, and fiber. Some diets do exist that recommend eating excessive protein, which in turn may harm the kidneys. A surplus amount of protein may dehydrate and stress your body. In many cases, this may also result in kidney failure (acute). This is because when the food is broken down after eating, the molecules of protein become larger, which is difficult to be processed by your kidneys.

- *Constipation* – If you follow severe dieting and that too for the long term, it may lead to constipation. It is that state when you may suffer from irregular or unusual bowel movements. Those who maintain a high-fat or low-fiber diet usually face this particular problem. Avoiding green leafy vegetables, fruits, and whole grains for a day or two may seem okay, but the situation becomes worse when this sort of diet is followed for a long period. The colon pulls in an extra amount of water, and thus stools tend to dry up and fail to pass smoothly, causing constipation.

- *Slowed metabolism* – First of all, you need to understand what metabolism actually is. It is the total quantity of calories that is necessary to fuel a person's body for performing the essential functions of life. If you eat more, your metabolism will increase and vice versa. The intake of calories decreases when you follow any typical diet, and thus, your metabolism slows down. It is true that in the beginning, you will start losing weight because of caloric restriction. But the scenario will gradually change with the passing of time. It is an indication that the pace of your internal metabolism slows down for matching the total number of consumed calories. People start 'pushing harder' regarding the restriction of calories as well as begin to exercise by using extra effort for reaching an energy balance that is negative. This again may lead to another phase of weight loss in the beginning and, after that, another plateau. This circle of pushing a bit harder than the previous phase continues, and after that, the result is equal to disappointment. In a maximum number of cases, the dieter becomes frustrated or irritated and tries to come out of the diet. He/she then goes back to their former eating habits, and the result is regaining weight.

- *Development of sagging skin* – The skin tends to become sagging and loose when a person loses weight with the help of dieting. It is because this particular sense organ is not capable of shrinking so rapidly as your body does. Sagging skin starts developing if you follow a diet for losing weight rapidly. Thus, a lot of proficient health experts provide a suggestion to focus on steady and slow weight loss. By doing so, your skin will get a lot of time for shrinking. Besides dieting, the loosening of skin is also dependent on various exercises that you practice. So, it is always better to consult or seek guidance from your gym instructor or fitness expert. He/she is the right person who will be able to create a perfect workout plan for you based on your diet or eating habits and lifestyle.

- *Causes menstrual problems* – If your weight keeps on fluctuating, it may also fluctuate your overall menstrual health and cycle. Rapid loss of weight is the result of severe dieting. When weight is lost at such a fast pace, a woman's body begins to shut down every single survival function that is not essential. This, in turn, has an adverse effect on menstrual cycles. Diets that involve the intake of low carb usually lead to irregular or unusual periods. If you plan to follow a keto diet and that too for a longer term, it may leave an intense impact on the menstrual cycle. The menstrual cycle is controlled by certain hormones like progesterone and estrogen.

If any changes occur in the production of these hormones, it gives rise to various menstrual problems. A lot of reliable studies exhibit that diet affects the hormone production of women. Nowadays, a maximum number of women tend to switch to an extremely rigid diet. But you might be shocked to know that it will disrupt the hormonal cycle in the worst manner. Sudden loss of weight, as well as weight gain, may have negative impacts on your menstrual health.

When a woman changes her diet suddenly, mostly restricting the consumption of certain foods for the fear of becoming fat, it may cause Amenorrhea. It is such a state when periods become absent or irregular for near about three to four months or in some cases more than that. It is caused because of sudden and too fast weight loss because of dieting, excessive exercise, etc. You may also suffer from irregularity in the menstrual cycle because of a diet that is rich in carbohydrates or a diet that lacks the necessary nutrition.

- *Causes headache* – To achieve weight loss effectively, a person usually intakes fewer calories than the amount burnt by his/her body. But when the required nutrition is not attained by your body, you may start feeling fatigued as well as experience dizziness and headaches. When an individual consumes an unbalanced diet or a diet containing insufficient calories, he/she may suffer from electrolyte imbalance. An imbalance of electrolytes means inappropriate potassium and sodium levels in the body, which in turn may lead to frequent headaches. Nowadays, a lot of people practice intermittent fasting to lose weight. It is necessary to fast for nearly twelve to fourteen hours to follow this form of dieting. This particular diet plan may not be suitable for all people because the requirement of each body is not the same at all. A person following this dieting plan may suffer from headaches because of a fall in blood pressure. Skipping meals or fasting for long hours also contributes to a low level of blood sugar, that is, Hypoglycemia. In such conditions, the dieter not only suffers from headaches but also dizziness and tiredness.

- *Altered mood* – You might be surprised to know that one of the worst side-effects of dieting is a negative change in your mood and energy. If you choose to practice dieting strictly, your body will not receive the appropriate amount of food. It may assist you in achieving your target weight loss, but it will affect your mood very badly. It is because of reduced levels of blood sugar as well as certain changes in the production of hormones. In general, an individual feels very tired because of a lack of energy if he/she consumes very little quantity of food. Tiredness often leads to a bad and irritable mood as well as frequent mood swings, depressions, etc. When you plan to follow a diet, you start eliminating various types of foods from your regular meal, and thus, your body will not get the essential nutrients properly. Lower levels of iron, zinc, magnesium, omega-3 fatty acids, vitamin D, and B vitamins are known to possess association with a decreased level of energy and worsened mood.

- *Affects the health of hair* – Almost all fad diets suggest the dieters consume very few calories. This means such diets won't add a sufficient quantity of vital nutrients to the body. It may result in malnourishment as well as tremendous loss of hair. The deficiency of both micro and macronutrients in a person's body may result in weak and dull hair. Poor nourishment leads to hair fall, hair breakage or damage, etc.

Thus, as you can see from the above points, dieting is indeed the biggest enemy of weight loss and your overall health.

Chapter 2: Figure Out the 'Why' Behind Your Goal of Losing Weight

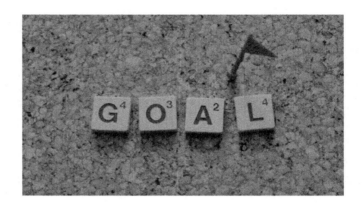

Losing body weight has become one of the most common tendencies among the majority of people nowadays. Initially, this tendency could be sighted among the youth as they get influenced by celebrity role models or fashion stars. But with time, this character trait has expanded itself among people of all age groups and also among all sections of society. So now it is indeed difficult to pinpoint any one reason as to why people want to lose weight. Some might do it because they want to look a certain way, while some might do it because they want to remain fit. Some might do it because their medical condition requires them to lose a certain amount to remain healthy, while others might not be happy with what they see in the mirror, and they want to get a certain body type. People can actually have various reasons which make them take direct and also indirect steps to lose weight.

There are numerous ways in which people try to lose weight these days. Some are healthy, and some are not, which can seriously cause damage. There are more than enough false and deceptive sights that sell medicines that help a person lose weight. These are extremely harmful; for the body and should never be taken by anyone. Some take the option of gyming and intense workouts. While some go for dieting, there are more than enough people who think that restricting their diet in certain ways will help them lose weight, and without knowing the basics, they blindly go for cutting all the necessary nutrients out of their bodies. While this might give an initial illusion of weight loss, restricting your body from getting all its necessary nutrients is extremely harmful. It only leads to your body getting into trouble by decreasing your immunity and making you ill.

The main aim for you to want to lose weight in the first place can be different but whether that is at all good for you or not is something that you have to consider first. Whether the reason for which you are trying to lose weight is at all healthy or not should be judged. It shouldn't be a mere psychological illusion or peer pressure among you when you clearly could have had other meaningful reasons. That is why even before you start taking any actions for losing weight, it is important for you to figure out whether you want it. As you start asking yourself all the necessary questions, you will surely understand what is best for you. Proceed only then. And if you do want to proceed with your weight loss program, it is imperative that you do something that will in no way harm your health and will be a natural healthy process. Let us then first understand why at all you need to know the 'why' behind the goal of losing weight.

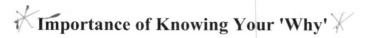

Importance of Knowing Your 'Why'

Ask yourself this extremely important question before you start your process of losing weight, and that is, "why do I want to lose weight?" before you do anything, knowing your reason for doing it comes first. It is often the most overlooked aspect in spite of being the most important one. You might randomly start doing it without knowing why and thereby, you are never prepared for the consequences that come with it. When you actually want to achieve something, in this case, a certain level of fitness, your "why" is crucial for your goal setting.

You might understand that once you lose weight, you will feel great physically and mentally, but you have also noticed that when you start working out, you cannot seem to continue it for a long time. You tend to give up after a few days for various reasons and excuses despite you wanting to lose weight. This might be because you are not really very clear about why you want to lose weight, and thus you lack enough motivation.

- *Knowing the 'Why' Helps With Fitness Goal Setting and Realistic Training Goals* – Unless you know exactly why you want to lose weight, the chances are that you will get confused among the various ways that are there for this purpose. What you need to understand is that not every method is suitable for everyone. We all are different individuals with different body types. Our bodies act differently under different circumstances, and we all have different dietary and fitness requirements, given whether or not we have any medical issues. So, just because something has worked for your friend does not mean it will work for you. There have to be different and practical ways that you need to take up which will be specifically fit and also useful for you in order for you to effectively lose weight. Unnecessarily pushing your body is definitely not a smart move to make. All your goals need to be realistic for them to actually work.

- ***Knowing Your 'Why' Will Tell You the 'How'*** – Unless you clearly know why you are doing something, you will not be clear in your mind as to how you need to do it. Keep in mind that no two people can use the exact same way to reach a similar goal. The way you will do something will have to be different from that of others. How you should do something and how long you should do it are very necessary and important questions that you need to find answers to if you want to lose weight properly. Your approach matters a lot. If your approach is not right, no matter what techniques you use, they will eventually be of very little value. So, ask yourself the question as to why you actually want to lose weight and then find out the way that is best suitable for you. You will need proper planning, adequate preparation, and a lot of hard work to get to your goal. If you have all these sorted, things will become far easier after that.

- *Knowing the 'Why' Gives You a Sense Of Purpose* – As I have mentioned before, when your reason for trying to lose weight is not clear to you, you tend to lose purpose. It is only natural for your mind to not back your body into doing something every day when the purpose is not really clear to it. That is the reason when you have a clear set of reasons in your mind; it becomes easier for your mind to hold on to that sense of purpose, and not only that, it also helps your body to push itself further for achieving that goal. For example, if you know that you need to lose a certain amount of weight for your medical conditions to improve, your mind will be determined to workout each day, and even if your body is tired, your mind will keep on reminding you as to why you need to lose weight. This will help increase the pace at which you take the various actions, helping you reach your goal faster.
- *Knowing the 'Why' Helps You in Understanding Yourself Better* – This is

something very interesting to consider. You see, many times, you do things without even giving them a proper thought. You might do it, as I have mentioned priorly, because of some new trend that you are following. In some cases, you might want to lose weight because you are not satisfied with yourself. So, when you ask yourself the important question, that is why at all you are doing this, you will get time to sit with yourself and know for sure what is going on in your mind. Is it something you are doing to bring a positive change in your life, or does this wish of yours have a negative connotation behind it? When you get answers to these questions, these answers will further open the forum for other very pertinent questions. For example, if this wish is backed by a negative attitude towards yourself, then why is it so? Did someone make you feel bad about yourself, or is there something you don't like about yourself? If that is the case, then what should you do to change it and better the situation for yourself? Such questions and answers are very helpful for you to know yourself better.

These are among the various reasons that will tell you the significance of the 'why.' It is your life, and at the end of the day, it falls on you to make it better for you to be happy. So when you have a solid purpose backed by a positive approach, it helps you become happier as a person and makes you feel what matters for you and what doesn't.

How to Figure Out the 'Why'?

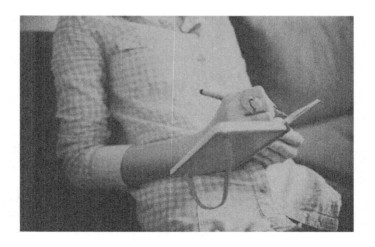

Now that you have a much better idea about why knowing the reason for what you are doing is so crucial, it is now time for you to understand how you can figure out the 'why'. Not everyone knows themselves properly. As ironic as it might sound, the reality is that though you might have a lot of idea about people around you and what they want and how they are, many a time you fail to give yourself that same importance, and what happens, as a result, is that you do not understand the reason behind your actions. That is why it might take you some time to figure out the actual reason behind your actions. Let us then see how you can figure out your 'why' easily.

Journaling	One of the best ways to know why you want what you want is to do some journaling. This is a method that is suggested even by professionals when you have a problem deciding something or coming to a decision.

	What you can try doing if you do not have the habit of journaling every day already is try assessing your feelings. Every day before going to bed, think about everything that happened that day and ask yourself what you felt when those things were happening. It doesn't matter how big or small these events are. Knowing how your mind works during a particular situation can give you a lot of insight into how you feel about things in your life. This will, in turn, help you to form better judgments and make

	practical decisions.
Make a List of Things That Matter	The next thing you can try doing if you want to understand the 'why' is to make a list of everything important to you. Be honest with yourself and make a list of things that are valuable to you and things that you want in life. When you write down this list, ask yourself why that is so. When you know what is important to you, along with why they mean so much to you, you will automatically have a much clearer vision regarding how you can plan out your actions for you to meet

	these goals and make these dreams a reality. The clearer these things are, the more concrete plans you will be able to make. Life will start seeming far less vague after that, and everything you do will have a concrete backbone to it.
Look Into the Past	It is important that you look in the past at times, giving you more incentives to try harder in the present for things you want. If I talk about losing weight, you might want to lose weight now because you want to go back to the weight you were a few years back. For

whatever reasons it might be, you might have put on weight, and you want to lose it now. Ask yourself what were those things in the past that used to give you happiness about that particular weight that you used to have. Ask yourself what the things that you used to do to maintain that weight were. Ask yourself what were those things in the past that used to help you maintain that weight. When you get the answers to these questions, you will see that it will act as t]an incentive in the present for you to try harder to

	lose your current weight and get back to the weight that you want to.
Look Forward to the Future	After you have taken incentives from the past, it is now important that you look forward to your future. I mean that you need to envision a future for yourself that will help you carry on in the present. You want to lose weight now because you want yourself to look and be a certain way in the future. Ask yourself what you will do when you actually achieve that goal. Ask yourself what changes you are

	anticipating in your way of life that will come in the future with this present change process. When you get these answers, you will see that the zeal with which you are working now will increase a lot. When you have a solid idea in your mind, it only gets easier for you to push yourself more and continue doing what you are doing now to get what you want in the future.
Decide on a Plan of Action	The final part of figuring out the 'why' starts when you initiate taking actual actions. Now that you have a fair idea about what

	you want and why you want it, it should not be too difficult for you to plan the actionable steps. When you want to lose weight, only wishing for it to happen and not really doing anything concrete will help you. You need to start taking immediate actions to bring out the desired results. Remind yourself constantly why you are doing it and make sure you choose steps that are flexible and yet effective. Do not for something that is completely out of your reach, as that will only add to your disappointment. If you

	get disappointed, that can make you distracted from your goal. Instead, take steps that you know you will be able to follow and make sure you do not let go of them. Taking the actions will automatically help you get a clearer idea about the entire thing and help you achieve your goal faster.

Common Psychological Blocks and How to Overcome Them

It is very common, and something that the majority of the people have already faced in life is a kind of mental setback when they have launched themselves in the weight loss journey and have found roadblocks. Mind you; it is not as easy as it sounds like to lose a lot of weight. For some, it comes fairly easily, but for most, it does not. It can take months and even years to lose weight. As humans, it is only natural for you to feel disheartened and have a sense of setback when that happens.

When you are taking action but not getting the desired results, you might be prone to giving up. But that should not be the case. There are ways to get over your psychological block so that even though you might feel bad, you can get over that feeling and start once again with renewed vigor. Let us look at some of the most common psychological blocks that you might face and also how you can deal with them.

Types of psychological blocks –

- *All-or-Nothing Attitude* – Psychologists use the term "cognitive distortion" to explain this condition. Many people out there face something like this where they tend to oscillate between extremes and not stick to a balance. What I mean by this is that either you stick to your meal plan or your workout routine completely, or you tend to fall off the hook. For starters, you go through your day doing the needful, but if someday due to any reason you fail to meet the requirements, that marks the beginning of your wayward journey. Missing the gym one day makes you not want to go for a week, probably. The right way for anyone is to maintain a balance where you have the confidence in yourself that even if you missed it for one day, you would be able to make up for it the next day. But when that does not happen, that rises to this condition of cognitive distortion.

- *Negative Body Image* – There is absolutely no harm in wanting you to look a certain way or be a healthier version of yourself. It is alright if you want to lose weight to maintain your figure. But what is wrong is when your desire to lose weight comes from the fact that you are extremely unhappy with what you see in the mirror. The problem occurs when your body image is negative and not one of positive improvement. For many people, a negative body image is attached to their lack of self-worth. You want to look a certain way because the way you look now is something that you are ashamed of, or it also might be that you are subjected to bullying. Here lies the problem. If you have a negative body image, it will invariably hinder your weight-loss process. Unless you are happy and have a positive outlook, it will cause issues.

- *Stress* – I am sure you have heard about comfort foods. Well, they are called so for a reason. It is a common characteristic for many people to resort to food and food items that they like when they are distressed or anxious. Food helps people, or rather that is what they think it does, to cope with anxiety. Now the problem that occurs as a result of this is that if you have the aim of losing weight, and if you are anxious about it, you might resort to eating unhealthy, and that will, in turn, increase your weight. This might continue as a vicious cycle if you do not understand what the actual matter is. It has also been seen that a person's food choices are likely to change when a person is anxious. You tend to consume food items with more sugar and higher calories when you are tense or anxious. That will invariably increase your weight. Stress can also cause further damage to your body as it produces more cortisol which is very potent to make you gain a lot of weight. It might so be the case that you are putting in a lot of effort to lose weight; you might be gyming, or you might be working out. But nothing will matter much, and your weight will remain the same, or it might even increase if you are stressed.

- **Depression** – Many types of research have shown that when a person is clinically depressed, they seem to gain a lot of weight due to various symptoms that depressions make a person go through. On the other hand, it has also been found out that for some people, depression leads to serious weight loss that is equally harmful to the body. If I take the first situation into consideration, when a person is clinically depressed, he\she might go through long episodes of sleeplessness or fatigue. Their mental state might lead them to resort to what they consider as their comfort foods. Another thing to consider is when a person is really worried and anxious about his\her weight, he\she might go into depression when they tend not to lose weight even after trying, and this depression, in turn, does not let their weight go down. Once again, it is like a vicious cycle. Depression then is really a potent cause of weight gain.

- *Childhood Trauma* – It has been proven after some research that those individuals who have suffered from any kind of childhood trauma like physical and psychological abuse or peer bullying, or sexual abuse are, by comparison, at a far higher risk of being obese when they grow up. As a defense mechanism to all the childhood trauma that they have gone through, many people develop very harmful food habits, and at the same time, some might resort to some kind of substance abuse which also can increase a person's weight. It is in no way indicated that if someone has unfortunately suffered from childhood trauma, they will struggle to maintain a proper weight. That is not the case. But it can be a situation where this happens.

These were some of the very common psychological issues that people go through, which might make them gain a lot of weight, and if not that, these issues can also make it extremely difficult for people to lose their existing weight. That being said, there are indeed many ways to overcome these psychological issues over time. If you are able to successfully overcome these psychological issues, you can very well lose weight and also maintain that, remaining healthy both physically and mentally.

Let us then look at some of the ways in which a person can effectively overcome such psychological issues.

- *Go For Small Changes* – The all-or-nothing mentality that I mentioned some time ago will invariably hinder your efforts from sticking to one particular strict weight loss plan. It will either make you work extra hard, or it will lead you to give up completely. That is the reason it is important that you trick your mind into believing that you can do it no matter what and take small steps going for small changes. Small changes might not feel too taxing at one go and what it does is benefit you immensely in the process. Make adjustments in your routine that will be comfortable for you and which you know you will follow until the end. Make sure these steps are flexible and not very overbearing. Ask yourself and also your fitness trainer such steps that are reasonable and effective. Most importantly, they are easily attainable. That way, neither will you feel guilty for missing out on your workout one day nor will you get too exhausted after doing it. There will be a good balance, and also it will be effective in slowly helping you get over your all-or-nothing attitude.

- *Communicate With Yourself* – This is a very pertinent fact that when you have a negative body image, it is only natural that you replay very negative messages to yourself throughout the day. Over time your mind takes these negative messages to be true, and that is the reason no matter what efforts you might be taking to lose weight, that doesn't have any effect. What this proves is that what messages you communicate to yourself can have a very crucial impact on your life. Use this opportunity to your advantage. When this can actually work, then instead of replaying negative messages to yourself, convey positive messages. Let me know that you are a confident and able person who is very much capable of maintaining proper weight and remaining fit. Your mind will start believing it, and very soon, you will be taking concrete steps to make this a reality.

Do not let your self-doubt be a negative force in your life. Instead, communicate with yourself and make sure you help yourself the most in your weight loss journey.

- *Maintain Sleep Hygiene* – Sleep is one of those things which your body needs in the appropriate amount to make sure all your bodily functions are working properly and that you are remaining healthy. A person who does not maintain proper sleep routines can very easily gain weight, making your bodily functions really twisted. You will be lethargic and perpetually tired if you are not sleeping well, and that can make your metabolism rate really slow. All these are potent causes for a person to gain weight. A lower metabolism rate does not let you digest your food well, and when that happens, you can easily fall ill and also gain weight. Lethargy and tiredness do not let you be actively involved in all the activities that you otherwise do. All in all, you need to make sure you are getting a proper amount of undisturbed sleep so that you feel fresh and enthusiastic about doing things and remaining mentally fit and healthy.

- *Seek Help* – Times have changed a lot, and nowadays, it is absolutely alright to seek professional help from mental health professionals if you think you need that. If you feel that there are certain psychological roadblocks on your path that you cannot overcome by yourself, it is alright to seek professional help from people who know what they are doing and who can give you a proper solution and suggest doable steps. These will help you first understand yourself better and know the root causes of why you are having these roadblocks in the first place. Secondly, it will help you understand what practical steps you can take to overcome these problems easily. When you want to lose weight for real, then you have to keep in mind that the road might not be very easy. But there will be much help for you on the way as well. All you need to do is take those help.

- ***Write the Issues Down*** – Another beneficial way to get over your psychological blocks is for you to write what you are feeling. Everyday fix a time for yourself where you will sit with yourself and your thoughts. Use this time to think about the reasons you think are stopping you from losing weight. Many times, people are in denial about the issues that they are facing. This denial makes it impossible to get to the root of the problem. Acknowledging that you might have an issue is the first step towards eradicating that issue. Write down what you think are your weaknesses and what are those problems that you are finding extremely hard to overcome. Understand yourself better and then take the next steps. The next step could be what you want them to be. You either take each issue and then try to solve it yourself, or you seek help from your friends and family or a professional. But when you understand the issues, you will know that things will get much easier for you.

Tips to Develop the Right Mindset

Losing weight can be done in various ways. Some are healthy methods that do not harm your body and your mind in any way. Those ways make sure your weight loss journey is a happy, painless and positive one. On the other hand, there are ways that are really unhealthy and harmful for you. Those methods put unnecessary pressure on your mind and your body, and they make you end up in an unhappy bad place which causes further problems in your life. These harmful methods can make you ill and put a stop to your weight loss journey. That is the reason it is absolutely imperative for you to know which steps to follow and which do not. You have to choose what is right for you. Thus I shall now mention some tips which will help you understand right from wrong and help you lose weight in a healthy and positive way.

- ***Clear Out All Your Misconceptions About Weight Loss*** – First things first. You need to revisit everything that you already know about weight loss. For all the time you have been trying to lose weight, you must have gathered a lot of information about the various techniques that help a person lose weight. In all probability, some of this information might be true and effective, while others might be wrong. You need to be absolutely sure which is which from the very beginning. Do not go on blindly following things because so and so have said so or because it has worked for someone else. Revisit everything that you have done and then see what has worked for you and what hasn't. Try and understand why they did not work out for you. Maybe they had been bad for your health or just not suited enough for you. Find out those reasons so that you don't make the same mistakes in the future.

- *Stop Using Opaque Food Containers* – This is an entirely psychological factor and immensely useful. You see, your brain has its own way of measuring things. When you eat your food from opaque containers, you naturally cannot see the amount that is there in the container. All you can see is the amount you bring up on the spoon to your mouth. This makes your brain feel that it has eaten a lot less than it actually has. On the other hand, if you eat from containers that are transparent, you can see the entire amount that is there in it, and no matter what method you are using to eat, that is your hand or your spoon or chopsticks, your brain will constantly remind you how much you have eaten and subsequently when you should stop eating further. When you use opaque containers, you tend to eat a lot more than what you are supposed to. That is the reason it is always advised to eat from transparent containers.

- *Stop Following a Diet* – Unlike what many may believe, dieting is not really a very good option for losing weight. Yet, it can help you to lose some initial kilos for the time being. But very soon your body's metabolism will get used to that and further impact of your diet will be lost. It is a common fact that people who start dieting tend to stop losing any more weight after losing a certain amount for some months. No matter what you do after that, it becomes almost impossible to lose any more weight. What you need to be is not restrict your mindset. Dieting does that to you. Dieting can make you get a very constricted mindset which hinders your weight loss procedure. You might feel that just because you are dieting, you can give up on working out and maintain other healthy habits. That will, in turn, stop your weight loss process. Instead, you can follow a plan that does not restrict you but helps you to have long-term goals that you can follow at your own pace.

- *Make Your Stomach Think That it is Full* – One of the most effective ways to lose weight is to trick your stomach into thinking it is full. You might have a habit of constantly snacking or munching on something mindlessly. This is really very harmful. You might be munching on sugary treats without even giving it any proper thoughts. What it does is lead you to gain a lot of weight in the process. So, when you see that you have this habit of constantly munching on something, munch on carrots or celery over sugary treats. Remove all such snacks from near you that can increase your weight. This will not let you have them even if you want to. Keep healthy snacks at hand so that when you cannot control your cravings, you have something healthy to eat, which will help you lose weight instead of gaining it.

- *Make Working Out a Fun Activity* – Working out can be really fun if you want to make it so. It is very natural for you to lose interest in working out and give up on gyming after a point if you are not really into a fitness mindset. That is why you need to find ways for yourself to make fitness a happy, fun, and exciting thing for you. When you start having real fun, it will only be a matter of time before you get into a proper habit of working out. Then it will not be a problem to lose weight anymore. You will happily work out and try to stay fit and healthy. Go for exercises that do not intimidate you and do not make you want to give up. There are countless workout options that help you lose weight. You don't need to do something that you are not comfortable with just because someone else is doing it. Take it at your own pace and do only that much that your health permits. When you get into the habit regularly, your body will automatically be able to take on more. You can then venture out to newer ways of weight training and weight loss procedures.

Losing weight can be really fun and doable if you want it to become so. It need not be as complicated and painstaking as it sounds. Whatever your reason for losing weight is, when you understand that and have the correct procedures in mind, it is only a matter of time before your body starts cooperating with you. Keep this truth in mind that you are beautiful just the way you already are. Your weight loss should not be due to something derogatory that someone might have said about your weight. You can do better without such people in your life. But if it is something that you are doing to make yourself feel good and become a healthy and fit person, go ahead and do it. You deserve to be happy in every way you want.

Chapter 3: Why is Exercise More Important and Effective Than Diet?

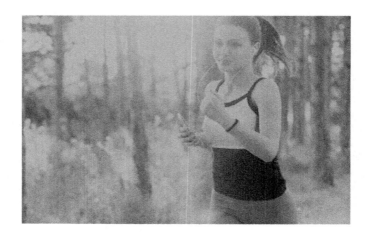

Do you feel very weak and tired after dieting for just a day? Do you feel like you have no energy to do any kind of work? Do you feel like sleeping all day long? If yes. Then you should stop dieting. Dieting is not for everyone; not every body type can deal with dieting. If you still keep doing it and avoid the problems you are having in your body because of dieting, you might fall severely ill. Thus, be careful about what weight loss option you are choosing and make sure that on the way to becoming fit, you do not end up becoming more unfit.

Most of the studies on dieting show that dieting also increases your food cravings, and you end up eating a lot more than you thought you would. Dieting can be really tough for a lot of people. Not eating enough food will not only make you feel tired and weak the whole day, but all irritated. You will get angry on small issues, and insignificant matters will also start bothering you. You will not be able to be truly happy and enjoy everything around you.

Dieting also stops you from socializing, and thus, you lose connection with your family and friends because of dieting. If you are not able to understand how that is possible, let me explain it to you. When your friends make a plan for dinner, you will start avoiding them because your dieting routine will get affected, and even if you think that you are going to go out with them and just order a salad to maintain your diet, you will end up eating what they have ordered and feel guilty about it immediately. You will also start avoiding family gatherings because even there, you will have to go and eat food that would affect your diet.

Experts believe that rather than concentrating on dieting a lot if you eat healthily and do exercises regularly, that would be much healthier for you. You would be able to see effective results really soon if you start exercising and eating clean. Eating clean and dieting are not the same thing. When you are dieting, you limit your calorie intake, but when you are eating clean, you just concentrate on eating good and healthy food and avoid eating junk. Cutting junk food out of your life and doing exercises regularly can give you more effective results.

Also, stopping yourself from eating all the things that you want to eat just because you are dieting will increase your hunger. Do not give yourself punishment for absolutely no reason. Eat whatever you feel like eating, just make sure that the quantity that you are eating is not a lot, avoid eating junk food and do your exercises regularly. This will keep you much healthier. Also, did you know that exercising and eating the right amount of food will also help you to deal with chronic diseases better because your body will have the power to fight back? For example, healthy people who eat their food without dieting and do exercise regularly have better chances of surviving cancer.

Thus, it is important that you do not waste your time trying to become fit by dieting; rather, use that time to do some exercises, which will give you a lot of benefits.

Is Exercise More Important?

The simple answer to this question would be yes. Yes, exercise is more important than dieting. Dieting might help you lose weight and reach your ideal weight really soon, but you will never become fit by following a particular diet. Exercise is much more important and necessary in your life. Doing some kind of exercise daily helps you to stay fit and healthy and also maintain a healthy weight and even lose weight in a healthy way. When you follow any particular diet, you limit the number of calories per day, but when you eat healthily and do exercise regularly, you are not just taking the right amount of calories that will provide you energy the whole day but also will help you to burn extra calories. When you exercise regularly, your physical exercises help you burn off a lot of calories, which helps you lose weight by creating a calorie deficit. A lot of research has shown that you can never lose weight properly by following a particular diet even though you put a limit on your calorie intake. Regular physical exercises are very important to maintain weight loss. Also, working out daily helps you to stay fit by reducing the risk of developing cardiovascular diseases and diabetes, which can be really bad for your health.

Do not try to just lose your weight, rather try to bring in an all-around good development in your body. Following a particular diet will only help you to lose weight, but exercising daily will not just help you to lose weight but also help you to become more fit. It has also been proven to reduce arthritis pain and also the risk of osteoporosis. Thus, doing some kind of exercise regularly will keep your body healthy, and you will be physically very strong.

But if you think that exercises just help you to reduce weight and stay healthy physically, then you might be totally wrong. Keep some time for yourself every day, and doing some kind of physical exercise also helps you to stay mentally healthy. It is proven that daily exercise reduces the risk of developing depression and also helps you to fight anxiety-related issues.

Also, did you know that if you keep following a particular diet, your body tends to lose the power of metabolism? When you limit your calorie intake, you are not just keeping yourself hungry all the time, but also you are making sure that your body loses the power of metabolism. Dieting can also lead to a nutritional deficit, and you might end up falling severely sick. Dieting has become a trend these days, but nobody actually knows what they are doing to their body. You make your own diet plan and think that eating less will help you to lose weight. But what you fail to see is that your chart has not been made by an expert who knows what amount of nutrition your body needs daily. Also, most people listen to what others eat daily and try to follow their diet, but they fail to understand that each body type is different, and the needs of each body are also very different.

Thus, without getting into this confusion and treating your body disrespectfully, it is better that you eat whatever you want, just make sure that it is healthy, and do some kind of physical exercise daily. You cannot even imagine how great that will be for your body.

Also, did you know that to lose your fat, you need to do some kind of physical exercise daily? Yes, to reduce your fat, you need to do some kind of physical exercise daily because exercises help you in burning that fat that dieting would never do. If you want to lose weight quickly, exercising is a must. Exercising daily helps you to increase your metabolism and thus you will end up burning more calories than you would by just following some kind of diet.

If you are someone who needs to go out and work daily, then dieting can never be your cup of tea. You are doing a lot of hard work, you might be traveling all day long, and that is never possible when you do not eat properly. Also, you will always be irritated and might not be able to give your 100% at your work just because you are distracted because of your hunger. Thus, it is very important for you to concentrate on eating properly first because that will help you to work better. Losing weight is very easy. Do not worry about it. Just take out half an hour before going to work or after coming home from work and do some cardio, and that will help you to lose weight. It will benefit you to be better at your work and also to lose weight and stay fit at the same time.

How Much Exercise Do You Need?

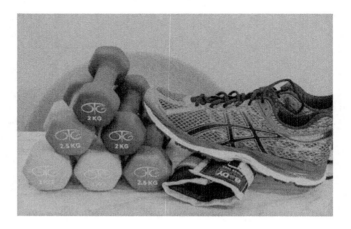

Doing exercises daily is very important. It is necessary to maintain healthy living, weight loss, and also maintaining a stable weight. But do you know for how long you should do any exercise or what is the correct time to do your exercises, so you get the most benefit from it? The basic concept is to burn more calories than you are intaking, and that will help you to lose weight. But how much exercise is needed to lose weight and stay healthy at the same time? Thus, here are a few guidelines provided by the experts that will help you to stay healthy and lose weight and also prevent you from gaining more weight in the future as well –

Daily exercises – Do not set an unachievable goal for yourself or a goal that you will not be able to achieve. Rather your goal should be realistic as that will help you to be motivated and will also push you to work harder. Aim at losing at least 1 to 2 pounds of weight per week. If you have to lose 1 pound of weight in a week, your daily calorie-burning aim should be 3500 calories. The physical activity that you choose totally depends on you. You can choose any exercise of your choice, and that will help you to lose weight and stay fit as well.

To lose 3500 calories per day, you could do these activities –

- You could run for 40 minutes daily.
- You could swim for 40 minutes daily.
- You could walk for 2 hours daily.
- You could cycle for 1 hour daily.
- You could also do intense aerobic classes for 1 hour daily.

If you can do any of the activities mentioned above, then you can lose weight and become fit and healthy at the same time.

Weekly exercises – Experts suggest that every person should do at least 30 minutes of exercise daily. It can be intense or light exercises depending on someone's needs, but 3o minutes of exercise daily is very important. Thus, 30 minutes of exercise daily means 150 minutes of exercise per week (it can be more than the given time as well). Some experts also suggest that 20 minutes of exercise three days a week is also enough if someone wants to avoid vigorous workout sessions.

But, the time totally depends on the amount of body fat that you want to reduce. If you are aiming at reducing a huge amount of body fat, then you will have to work a bit hard every day, but if your aim is to maintain your weight and be fit at the same time, then you can do less intense workouts. Remember that your body type is different, and thus, the exercises for your body will also be different. It depends on your age, sex, weight, and activity level as well. Thus, choose your exercise pattern carefully.

Make sure that you are creating the right routine for weight loss –

If you are someone who does not have a lot of time, then how will you design your workout routine so that you can reach the goal that you have set for yourself? How will you understand that the goal that you are setting for yourself is achievable if your workout routine is set on a daily basis or on a weekly basis? To find the answer to these questions, you will need to understand when and how much time you will be able to invest in your workout schedule.

Shorter workout – If you are someone who has the time to work out daily, then it is one of the best things you can do. If you can invest 20 to 30 minutes daily and work out properly, then you can lose weight easily. Exercising daily will also help you to stick to it, and this will become a good habit. The best way you could do your exercise daily is to wake up early and do the amount of exercise you were about to do, burn off that calorie that you were supposed to burn, and you will be done for the day. Doing exercises early in the morning will also help you to feel motivated the whole day, and your day will also be a productive one. You could also go to the gym while coming back from work directly every day, and that will help you to achieve the goal that you have set for yourself every day.

Work out fewer days in a week – We all know that working out daily can be next to impossible for most people. These days, people are really busy in their lives, and making time to work out every day can be really tough. That also does not seem realistic as well. You might be really busy with your work or with your family, and giving time to these things in your life is also very important. Thus, you can very well choose to work out fewer days in a week and still be fit. For example, you can work out for 45 minutes two days a week and 60 minutes on the weekend. This will be enough for you to stay fit and achieve your goal. The other option you have is that you could do a double workout on days when you have time. For example, if on a particular day you do a lot of walks, you could wake up early and go for a morning walk or jog and then in the evening you could also hit the gym or do any other kind of exercise. Even so, the method will help you to stay healthy and lose weight. Remember, your main aim should be to build an exercising habit, and if you push yourself in the first few weeks, you will find yourself automatically motivated after that. Also, once you start losing weight, you will automatically feel motivated and work hard to fulfill your workout goal.

A mixture of both – Your workout does not need to be either daily or weekly; it can be a mixture of both as well. Your workout routine should be the best suited for you. Your main aim is to lose weight by burning calories, so it does not matter how you are working out; rather your workout matters. Your workout should suit your body type. Also, once this becomes your habit and your fitness level has increased, you can aim to burn higher calories and challenge yourself every now and then. Working out every now and then and doing an intensive workout daily is much better than doing dieting as that might make you lose weight at first, but you will be losing your metabolism power, and also your body will lack a lot of essential nutrients. Remember that dieting cab has adverse effects on your health as well. Thus, be careful about which weight loss method you are choosing for yourself and remember your priority - is it to just lose weight or is it to lose weight by being healthy and fit at the same time? Thus, think about it and make the right choice.

Common Exercises to Lose Weight

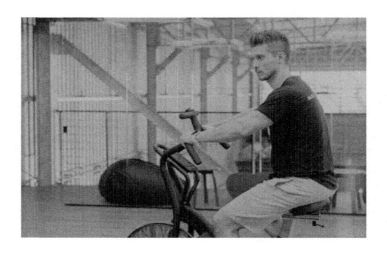

Exercises of all kinds help you to stay fit, but when your main aim is to lose weight along with staying healthy, then you will need to work a bit harder and concentrate on exercises that are effective for weight loss. Here is a list of various types of exercises that will help you to lose weight –

HIIT (High-Intensity Interval Training) – Losing weight includes both healthy eating and exercising. You will have to burn off more calories than you are intake, and HIIT helps you to reach your desired weight easily. This particular exercise pattern is a combination of cardio and strength training. Cardiovascular exercises increase your heart rate, and that helps you to lose weight most effectively. Experts say that you need 600 minutes of cardio workout every week and that your workout should have three splits – 20 minutes of walking in the morning, 20 minutes of walking after a lunch break, and 20 minutes of high-intensity workout at any time of the day. Strength training exercises do not do fast results. Thus you will have to be patient to see the results of it. It does not just help you to lose weight, but also it can boost your metabolism and help you to build lean muscle mass.

Here are some cardio and HIIT exercises that will help you to lose weight –

Low-Intensity Cardio	If you are a beginner, you will not be able to do high-intensity workouts at first. You will need to train your body first, and for that, you need to start with low-intensity workouts. Beginners mostly have physical limitations but do not worry; the low-intensity workout will also help you to burn off fats and help you to lose weight. Low-intensity workouts like swimming, jogging, power walking, and aerobics can help you a lot to lose weight. On

days when you have some extra time, you could also go for a bike ride and enjoy your workout session. Remember that you will have to start slowly and then gradually increase the intensity of your exercises, and you will get adjusted to the new routine in no time. For example, you could start with 60 minutes of low-intensity workout five days a week at first, and then as you become used to this exercising routine, you could bring change in it and make it more intense by adding some weight to your hands

	while jogging.
Jumping Ropes	It is also one of the best workouts that will not just help you to lose weight and stay fit but also will help you to improve the cognitive function of your body. This form of cardio is very effective as it increases your heart rate and helps you to burn 1300 calories every hour. The process in which it should be done is that you should start your warm-up with 8 to 10 jumps and then increase your intensity and jump for about 11 to 12 minutes continuously without

	stopping for even a second. After completing that, you can rest for 30 seconds and then again continue with it. If you are able to do three sets of this daily or on the days when you are exercising, that will be enough for you. If you are a beginner, then you can also jump with one leg so that it becomes a bit easier or low-intensity for you, and you can also keep switching your legs.
Burpees	You could also do burpees as that helps you lose weight and become fit in a very short time. Burpees are

basically the combination of 3 exercises; they are – squats, jumps, and then pushups. When you combine these three workouts, it helps you a lot to lose weight, and it is very effective as well. It helps you to burn a lot of fat as this particular exercise includes the movement of your whole body. This particular exercise also helps and serves as muscle training for your legs, chest, and core. The best and most effective way to do it is to do it ten times without stopping in about 30 seconds and

	repeat it for 5 minutes.
High-Intensity Interval Training (HIIT)	I am sure that you have heard about this type of workout. This is one of the most popular types of workout, and the reason why it has gained so much popularity is that it helps you to burn a lot of calories in just a few minutes. This particular workout has the ability to maximize your fat loss and calorie burn. This particular workout is a combination of excessive and intense workouts for some time that will increase your heart rate a lot, then followed by 15 seconds of rest. This exercise is

	basically designed for people who do not have much time but still want to stay fit and healthy and lose weight at the same time. This exercise helps you to work out for a very little amount of time and makes sure that you burn off a lot of calories during that time. This exercising pattern is so intense that it makes sure that you keep burning off calories hours after you have completed your workout. For example, you can do butt kicks for 45 seconds without stopping and then take a rest for 15 seconds.

	Then move on to jumping lunges for another 45 seconds and then take rest for 25 seconds again. Move on to burpees after your 15 seconds of rest and do it for another 45 minutes and after completion, take rest for 15 seconds. Repeat these exercises and this pattern for around 20 minutes, and that will be enough for you. You can also include other movements like mountain climbing and squats in this routine. Or, you could also complete your HIIT workout on a treadmill if you have one. You can do warm-up for 5

	minutes and walk at a slow to medium pace during this time. Next, move on to high-intensity speed for 1 minute and again slow down the speed for 30 minutes. Keep doing this and try to do at least ten sets of this exercise pattern, and you will be done for the day.

Here is a list of some strength training exercises that will also help you to stay fit and lose weight –

Kettlebell Swings	This strength training exercise involves the movement of your whole body and will increase your heart

rate. This exercise also helps you to increase the strength of your legs and hands, and thus, in the end, you also develop a strong core. But as I have mentioned earlier, strength training does not show its results easily or very fast; you will need to work out every day and only then will you be able to see the results after a few months. You will have to start by holding the kettlebell with both hands and swing it for 20 seconds. Next, you will have to take a rest for 8 seconds and then continue with it again. Complete eight sets of

	it daily, and you will see the results in a few months. Experts recommend that you lift it faster as that boosts your heart rate and thus helps you to lose weight.
Pushups	If you want to make your core strong, then pushup is one of the best exercises that you can do. It does not involve any equipment. Rather you will just have to use your upper body strength to do this exercise. Thus, it also helps in muscle mass building of your upper body, including your arms. If you are someone who is new to

	pushups, at first, it will seem to be really tough, and you might also feel like giving up, but do not give up. If you are a beginner, take it slow, start with three sets, and each set should consist of 10 pushups. Then take a rest for 60 or 90 seconds in between each set. Once you get used to this, keep increasing the number of sets as that will help you to keep improving your strength.
Lunges	Lunges might seem to be really easy and not very hard to do, but once you start doing it, you will surely be able

	to understand how effective it is. You have the option of doing front lunges and back lunges, or you can even do a mixture of both. To make it more difficult, you can also add a weight plate and then do your lunges. This will make it more challenging, and you will be able to lose weight and be fit easily. Make sure that each set consists of 8 to 12 lunges for each leg.
Step-Ups	Step-up is also considered one of the most important and great strengthening exercises that will help you increase your core

	strength, and the stability of your body will also improve. This strengthens your leg and also your lower back muscles. For doing this exercise, you will need a small step height and then as you become more comfortable and make progress, keep increasing the height to around 24 to 30 inches. This exercise should consist of 5 sets, each consisting of 5 to 10 step-ups. If you want to challenge yourself and lose more weight, then you can add weight to it like; for example, you could hold a dumbbell or a kettlebell

	and do the step-ups. This will help you to accelerate your heart rate as well.
Deadlifts	If you are someone who has the idea that deadlifts only help in muscle building, then you are completely wrong. Yes, deadlifts help in building your muscles and also make your core really strong but also, it helps in reducing excessive fat of both the lower and upper body. Experts advise that you focus on repeating the lifts rather than increasing the weight you are lifting if your main aim is to lose weight. For

	example, you can do three sets, and each set should comprise 10 to 20 deadlifts. Do this for a few months, and you will be able to see great results. You will not just lose weight but also feel a lot stronger.

Yoga – You might think that yoga does not help in weight loss, rather it helps you to stay fit and maintain a healthy weight. But that is where you are absolutely wrong. The popular belief about yoga is totally wrong. Yoga can help you to lose tons of calories and promote weight loss if you know the correct method of doing it. Choosing your asanas is also very important. If you have made the right choice and chosen the right kind of asana, then you will lose weight in no time. Yoga is that kind of exercise that not only helps you to lose weight and keep you fit but also helps you to attain mental peace and stability. It reduces your stress, anxiety, and depression as well. The benefits of doing yoga every day are huge.

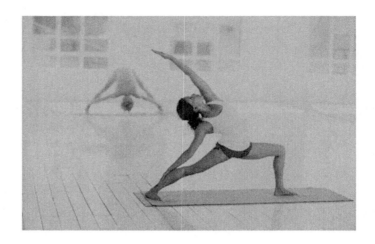

Here are some anas that will help you to lose weight and attain your goal quite easily –

Utkatasana or the Chair Position	In this position, you have to sit in an imaginary chair position by bending your knees and pushing your pelvis. This will directly affect your stomach and will help

	you to reduce your extra belly fat. Try to hold this position for some time and while holding the position, try inhaling and exhaling. Keep doing this asana at least ten times and each time, try to hold it for a longer time period.
Trikonasana or the Triangle Pose	We all know that yoga asanas are mostly simple, yet they are very effective. To achieve this position, you will just have to stand straight with your legs 2 feet apart from each other. Next lift both the hands sideways and bring one of the hands-down and

	touch your feet, bend your torso and the other hand should be pointed towards the ceiling. Hold this pose for at least 20 seconds before changing it and doing it on the other side. This simple yoga asana has been proven to be very effective and helps in reducing fat.
Virabhadrasana 2 or Warrior 2	This is yet another very simple yet very effective asana that helps in weight loss and staying fit. To achieve this pose, you will have to stand with your feet wide apart from each other and your hands by your side. Take a step and

	bend your knee to a 90-degree angle and turn your other foot at a 15-degree angle. Now lift both the arms sideways to your shoulder level with your palms facing towards the ceiling. Try to hold that position as much as you can and also try to bring your pelvis down while you are doing it. Repeat it on the other side as well.
Dhanurasana or Bow Position	As the name suggests, for achieving this position you will have to make your body look like a bow. For this, you will have to lie on the ground on your stomach and make sure

	to place your feet apart. Now try to hold your feet with your hands and put it as much as you can. Pull it in a way so that your legs and chest are off the ground and only your belly touches the ground. Try to keep your face straight and hold the position for some time. Make sure that your body is tight while you are doing this asana. This will help you to reduce your body fat tremendously.
Setu Bandha Sarvangasana or Bridge Position	As the name suggests, when you achieve this position, your body will look like a bridge. To achieve this

	position, you will first need to lie down on the ground on your back. Now press your feet on the floor and lift your body. Make sure that only your feet and your head are touching the ground. Now try to touch your feet with your hands and lift your chest as much as you can. Also, force your butt muscle to push your hip higher. Hold this position for some time, and you will become fat to fit in no time.
Bhujangasana *or* ***Cobra Pose***	This is also very effective in reducing your belly fat. To achieve this position,

	you will have to lie on your stomach and try to keep your feet as close to each other as you can. Now bring your palms near to your shoulder and lift your body as much as you can. Only your legs should be touching the ground. Your stomach and chest should be lifted upwards. Also, try looking at the ceiling. Hold this pose for some time and repeat it at least ten times daily. This will not just reduce your belly fat but also be a great exercise for your hip.
Navasana or the Boat	In this pose, you will

Pose	have to make your body look like a boat that is flowing in the water. To achieve the position, you will have to sit on your mat with your legs placed on the floor. Try to lift your legs from the floor and also try to bring your shin parallel to the floor. Your whole body should be resting on your butt, which means the only part of your body that should touch the ground is your butt. Hold your legs uptight so that your body looks like a 'V.' Also, put your arms forward. Hold the pose for some time, and this will make your core strong

	and build your core muscles as well.

Aerobic Exercises – If you want to lose weight the proper way, you can engage yourself in any exercise you want. Aerobics is one of the exercises that help you to lose weight and become fit. Also, if you want to lose weight fast, then choosing aerobic would be a good option for you. Aerobics exercises include cycling, jogging, running, power walking, dancing, Zumba dancing, swimming, etc. All these exercises will increase your heart rate and help you to burn off that extra fat really quickly. It is a much better option than dieting, and thus, you will be more fit and be able to control your body weight easily.

Other than doing the exercises mentioned above, you can also try to be active all day long by doing simple things. This will keep your body moving and help you to lose weight as well. These are –

- If you are watching some show on the tv, walk in the room during the commercial breaks or even when you are talking to someone over the phone.

- Do not use your car to go to someone nearby, rather walk and go there if you have time.

- Do not use the elevator, rather use the stairs to climb up.

- You can also use some fitness tracker apps to track your daily activity, as that will keep reminding you to be active if you have been resting for a long time.

- You can also get off the bus at the stop that comes before your destination and walk the rest of the way.

- Also, while doing your house chores or cooking, put on some music that will get your work done really soon and also encourage you to dance a bit and do some physical activity as well.

- You can also take your dog for a walk every now and then.

Thus do not run behind losing weight. Losing weight should not be the only goal in your life. It is true that when you lose weight, you keep away from a lot of diseases, but if you try to lose weight the wrong way, that is by dieting, then there is a high chance that your body will lack all the necessary nutrition and you will become very weak and fall sick in the process. Thus, your aim should be to become fit and lose weight the correct way. Concentrate on eating healthy food, avoid eating junk, and do a lot of exercise, and in no time, you will become much healthier and also lose weight and achieve the goal that you have set for yourself.

Chapter 4: Little Habits That Can Make Big Changes in the Long Run

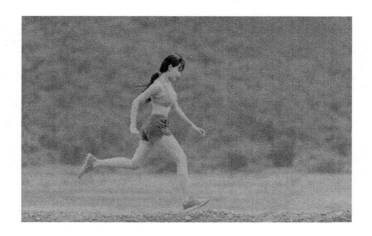

Are you in the group of those people who hold a firm belief that the one and the only way of losing weight is following a strict diet? If your answer is a big yes, then this book is the perfect one for you because it will show you how diet can actually be detrimental, as we have already discussed in Chapter1. Here you will get to know that the belief that you have been holding for so long is not the actual case when it comes to weight loss. Sustainable and healthy weight loss can be achieved perfectly with the help of very minute changes or habits to the existing lifestyle. You might feel attracted by noticing the review of certain diets that promise to help in shedding pounds. The truth is that if you follow such diets, you may lose weight very quickly, and that is helpful in giving you a successful feeling. But the sad part is that your lost weight will return at a quick pace along with some more additional pounds.

Journeys related to weight loss are not at all super easy and quick. The time has come for you to throw away certain wrong beliefs regarding strict dieting and weight loss. A maximum number of diets involve calorie restriction. You need to understand one fact very clearly that every single individual possesses a unique body, and the reaction towards calorie restriction is also different. A certain amount of calorie restriction might prove to be fruitful for your friend. But that does not mean the result will be the same in your case too. You must not feel disheartened for that and also not lose hope. Losing weight is actually possible even if you do not cut off the intake of calories from your daily meals.

So, think twice before you begin torturing your entire body just for the sake of losing weight. You need to start believing that weight loss is possible even by ceasing dieting. Restrictive dieting provides an effect that is termed as yo-yo effect, which means you lose weight and gain it again. This is a never-ending cycle. Numerous effective ways, or you may say habits, do exist with the help of which an individual may lose weight and that too without involving dieting. You just need to start believing in yourself and proceed to follow little habits that can bring about huge changes in the long run. Here you will get to know about a few habits that will assist in healthy and consistent weight loss. So, have a look!

Sleep Adequately

Almost all people know that sleep is good for health as it is helpful in re-energizing the body for further activities. Besides this, sleep has healthy connections with an individual's weight. If you do not allow your mind and body to rest sufficiently, it will leave a negative effect on your weight. While you spend sleepless nights, your body begins to cook up an ideal recipe for gaining weight. A lot of individuals might get shocked to know that quality and adequate sleep is an integral element of any healthy weight loss plan. It is quite unfortunate that a huge number of individuals are not sleeping for the required quantity. As per some authentic studies, almost thirty percent of adults sleep for less than 6 hours for a countless number of nights. Well, interesting evidence is that adequate sleep is one of the missing factors for those people who continuously struggle to lose weight. Several reasons are there that will help you in understanding the reason behind losing weight with the help of enough sleep.

Fewer hours of sleep increase a person's appetite by disrupting the perfect balance of those hormones that are meant for controlling appetite. Two hunger hormones, namely leptin, and ghrelin, are responsible for giving hunger signals and shaping a person's appetite. The latter one is that hormone whose duty is to inform you when you should eat. On the other hand, the former hormone gives a signal so that you get to know when to cease eating.

Ghrelin levels reduce during the night as your body does not need to produce a huge quantity of energy when you sleep in comparison to the time when you stay awake. The level of leptin escalates as it informs the control center of your body, that is, the brain, that it is not necessary to bring about hunger at night. So, if you do not get enough sleep, the ghrelin level in your system will rise up a lot. Your body will start assuming that it is hungry and feel the urge to intake more calories. Besides this, an inadequate amount of sleep results in the reduction of leptin levels. This, in turn, makes a person feel that he/she is feeling hungry. Thus, the end result of less leptin and more ghrelin leads to weight gain. Another hormone called cortisol also increases if an individual is deprived of sufficient sleep. This particular stress hormone may increase your appetite too.

A trustworthy study including almost a thousand people states that those who sleep for a short duration possess 15.5% lower levels of leptin and 14.9% higher levels of ghrelin than those individuals who sleep for an optimum duration.

Poor sleep is also linked with a higher BMI or body mass index as well as weight gain. Now, you might think that sleep requirements vary from one person to the other. It is true. But speaking in general terms, certain research regarding this matter has noticed a change in weight when individuals sleep for less than 7 hours per night. An important review stated that a short duration of sleep boosts the chances of being obese by fifty-five percent in adults and eight-nine percent in children. In addition to all these, a lot of sleeping disorders, such as sleep apnea, tend to worsen because of weight gain. It is a monstrous cycle that is very difficult to escape. Poor sleep leads to weight gain and this, in turn, hampers the quality of sleep even further.

Individuals who get less quantity of sleep have a tendency to consume more calories than usual. An interesting study was conducted for which a total number of twelve men were included. The participants were not permitted to sleep for more than four hours. When they slept for the mentioned duration, they consumed about 559 calories on average the next day, in comparison to those days when they slept for almost seven to eight hours. This escalation of calorie intake may be because of poor choice of foods and increased appetite. Some other studies on sleep deprivation revealed a fact that a great part of the extra calories is usually consumed after dinner in the form of late-night snacks. Other than that, lack of proper sleep may also increase the intake of excess calories by affecting a person's ability to control or balance his/her portion sizes.

The bottom line is that quality sleep is one of the essential parts of maintaining weight and controlling weight gain. Less amount of sleep changes the manner your body gives response to foods. In the beginning, your appetite will increase, and you will not be able to resist the temptation of eating more and controlling portions. Your responsibility is to break this vicious cycle. The fewer hours of sleep you get, the more pounds you will gain; the more you gain weight, the more difficult it will become to sleep. So, if you establish healthy sleeping habits, then you will be able to maintain your body weight. Now, here are some of the tips that will assist you in ensuring that you receive enough quantity of quality sleep.

Try drinking one glass of milk just before you go to sleep every night. Milk consists of an amino acid named tryptophan. This specific amino acid will help you in relaxing when you try to sleep. Another way of controlling sleepless nights is by avoiding all sorts of caffeinated drinks after three in the afternoon. It is because caffeine is a type of stimulant and results in the disruption of good sleep. Moreover, caffeine has the capability of staying inside your system for almost five to six hours. If you are willing to lose weight by bringing certain changes in your daily habits, then you must change your dinner time. Instead of practicing late dinner, you will get fruitful results if you have early dinner. If you take a very late dinner, your system will get stimulated instead of calming down. This, in turn, will decrease the chances of being successful in terms of weight loss.

Healthy sleep can also be achieved by drinking plenty of water throughout the entire day. You must not worry at all as excess water will not be retained by your body. Your task is to check that you stay hydrated no matter how busy your schedule is.

Switching off all the electronic gadgets after 10 p.m. also works wonders in getting you a long duration of soundless sleep. The light that is emitted by the screens of computers, laptops, mobile phones, TVs, and tablets hampers melatonin production. Melatonin is a hormone that controls the circadian rhythm or awake or sleep cycle of a person. Turning out all the lights in your bedroom also ensures good sleep. Darkness provides a clue to your body for releasing this sleep hormone naturally. Light is known to suppress the production of this hormone.

Another tip that might help you in getting a sufficient amount of sleep is creating a certain bedtime ritual. You need to understand one fact that bedtime is not at all the time for tackling big issues. Your bedtime rituals may include taking a warm bath, reading romantic storybooks, meditating while listening to mind-calming or relaxing music, etc. You must learn to adapt to various ways of reducing your stress level. Chronic stress leads to insufficient quantity of sleep as well as weight gain. It even includes excessive eating for coping with unfavorable emotions. A sufficient duration of quality sleep can also be achieved if you follow the habit of going to bed early. It is because individuals who have a tendency to go to bed very late at night may intake more calories. It increases the risk of gaining more weight.

Thus, the time has come for making such little changes in your sleeping habits so that you can lose weight and stop regaining more. If you are determined to practice the above-mentioned steps, then start from today onwards and do not wait for tomorrow.

Consume a Good Deal of Protein

Yes, protein! It is the one and the only nutrient that assists in losing weight consistently as well as gaining an attractive-looking body. Foods that are rich in protein are well known for the property of losing weight. You need to include such foods in your breakfast for attaining weight loss quickly and in a healthy manner. Protein can reduce hunger and let you feel full, which, in turn, is beneficial in restricting the intake of calories. It is because protein has the capacity of affecting certain hormones that deal with your hunger as well as fullness, namely GLP-1 and ghrelin.

A person's overall body weight is regulated by the brain, especially the hypothalamus. While your brain determines how much and when to consume food, it deals with various kinds of information. The hormones that exhibit a change in feeding patterns provide essential signals to an individual's brain. If your body experiences a higher quantity of protein intake, then it elevates the satiety levels of hormones that reduce appetite, namely peptide YY, cholecystokinin, etc., whereas it decreases the level of ghrelin which is the hunger hormone. By substituting fats and carbs with protein, you decrease ghrelin and boost the level of various satiety hormones. It decreases hunger, which is the most important reason behind protein helping in weight loss. It provokes a person to consume fewer calories, and that too automatically.

The foods that consist of this essential nutrient help hasten your metabolism. The metabolism that can work efficiently eases the procedure of losing weight. If your metabolism is healthy, it will assist you in burning more calories. You might get surprised to know that a huge quantity of calories is necessary for metabolizing protein when compared to carbohydrates. So, if you add a sufficient amount of protein-rich food to your daily meals, it will assist you in losing weight, even without intentional calorie restriction. After consuming food, some quantities of calories are utilized for digesting as well as metabolizing food. It is often referred to as TEF or thermic effect of food. Indeed, all types of sources may not agree with the perfect figures. But protein possesses a thermic effect (20-30%) which is a little more in comparison to fat and carbs, having a thermic effect (0-3%) and (5-10%), respectively. If you consider the 30% thermic effect of protein, it means that one hundred calories of this nutrient simply result in a total number of seventy usable calories. In simpler words, about 30% of calories in protein get burned when your body performs functions such as digesting as well as metabolizing it.

An authentic study including obese or overweight women was conducted. In that study, it was observed that the women who ate eggs at the time of breakfast consumed less quantity of calories during lunch hours compared to others who included grains in their breakfast. Besides this, those who had eggs consumed very few calories almost throughout the entire day as well as during the duration of the following 36 hours.

You might also feel quite content to know that protein possesses the capacity of reducing appetite and thus lets a person consume fewer calories than usual. This particular nutrient decreases appetite and hunger through certain different mechanisms. It may automatically lead to a decline in the intake of calories. You will end up consuming fewer calories and that too without the need of controlling portions consciously or counting calories. Innumerable studies related to this matter have revealed or concluded that when an individual elevates his/her protein intake, he/she will start consuming fewer calories. This theory functions on the basis of both meal-to-meal and also a continuous day-to-day decrease in the intake of calories when the intake of protein is kept elevated.

Another convincing and reliable study reveals that protein possessing 30% calories leads people to drop down their calorie consumption naturally by 441 calories every single day. Isn't it a huge amount? Thus, by now, you might have realized that diets that are high in protein not only possess metabolic benefits but also have appetite advantage. It helps in cutting down calories much more easily than diets that are low in protein.

Consuming a good deal of protein reduces cravings as well as cuts down the desire to consume snacks late at night. Truly speaking, late-night cravings are regarded as the worst enemy of all people who are trying to lose their extra weight. A lot of people who tend to put on weight get food cravings during the night hours, so they consume snacks in the evening hours. These calories get included above the total amount of calories that they consumed in the entire day. It is quite interesting to know that protein may have a strong effect on cravings and the desire to snack late-night. The first meal of the day, that is, breakfast, is considered to be the essential time for loading protein into your system. One study including teenage girls exhibited that consuming a breakfast that included a high amount of protein reduced cravings quite significantly. Such small changes prove to be helpful in sticking to healthy eating from the very beginning of the day.

This essential nutrient can work on dual sides of the equation 'calories in versus calories out. Protein decreases the intake of calories as well as boosts the calories out. Hence, it is not at all surprising to view that diets that are rich in protein result in loss of weight and that too without restricting portions, calories, carbs, or fats intentionally. In a study including a total number of nineteen individuals who were overweight, escalating the intake of protein to thirty percent calories resulted in a huge drop in the intake of calories. The participants of this study lost nearly eleven pounds of weight on an average within a duration of eleven to twelve weeks. You need to keep in your mind that those people only included protein-rich foods in their diet and did not restrict anything intentionally. A majority of studies exhibit that diets that are rich in protein end up in vital weight loss. Consuming protein-rich foods is even connected with less belly fat, one of the most harmful fats accumulated around organs causing diseases.

People who follow different types of diet may lose weight for the time being, but a maximum number of them regain the weight. Another interesting fact is that a higher quantity of protein intake may also assist in preventing the regaining of weight. So, this highly essential nutrient helps in losing extra pounds and proves to be extremely helpful in preventing its return for the long term. Now, you might be wondering about how to include more quantity of protein into your regular meals. Well, you need not worry at all as boosting the intake of protein is very much simple. You just need to consume a greater quantity of foods that are rich in protein. Here you will get to know about a few foods that consist of protein.

- *Fish*: Sardines, salmon, trout, haddock, tuna, etc.
- *Legumes*: Chickpeas, kidney beans, lentils, etc.
- *Eggs*: Almost all types
- *Meat*: Turkey, pork, chicken, lean beef, etc.
- *Dairy*: Yogurt, cottage cheese, cheddar, mozzarella, Swiss cheese, Parmesan cheese, Greek yogurt, milk, etc.
- *Nuts*: Almonds, cashews, pistachios, etc.

Consuming protein is indeed very simple if you think about it casually, but integrating it into your nutrition plan and life may seem to be difficult. For easier inclusion, you may take the help of a nutrition or calorie tracker in the initial stage. So, if you are willing to get a better appearing body as well as fat loss, protein becomes the ruler of all other nutrients. There is no necessity of restricting any single thing for getting the benefits of a larger protein intake. It is simply about adding such foods to your daily meals. It is also an effective strategy of preventing obesity, not those that are used temporarily for losing fat.

Drink More Water Regularly

Water is life as well as an essential helper of losing weight. An estimated percentage of thirty to fifty-nine percent of US citizens, mostly adults, who have the intention or desire to lose weight increase the quantity of water consumption. A lot of reliable studies exhibit this theory that consuming plenty of water has the benefit of both weight maintenance and weight loss. Apart from these, hydration is also important for various other factors that have a great impact on digestion, the functioning of muscles, etc. Here you will get to learn about some of the reasons why water consumption in an adequate amount assists in losing extra pounds.

Whenever you feel hungry, the first impulse is to search for food and consume it as fast as possible. An individual may also assume that he/she is hungry when it is nothing other than thirst. Thirst is also generated by slight dehydration, and the brain thinks it to be hunger. You will be able to reduce appetite by intaking water if, by chance, your body has less quantity of water and no calories. Thus, water is treated as an appetite suppressant (natural).

Drinking plenty of water may promote satiation as it has a tendency of passing through your system at a quick pace by stretching your stomach. Thus, the message is sent to the brain that signals fullness. A lot of proficient and experienced nutritionists also suggest drinking a little bit of water just before eating your food as it may assist in reducing the food intake. This particular theory is supported by authentic research. One such research included some individuals who drank two glasses full of water just prior to a meal. It is reported that those people ate almost 22% less food than those people who avoided drinking water before having a meal. How much water must be consumed before sitting down for a meal to suppress appetite? Now, this question might be poking your brain after going through this theory. Almost two cups of water are enough to fill up your stomach so that your brain is able to register a certain amount of fullness.

Another study that was conducted in the year 2014 included fifty females who were overweight and willing to lose weight without following a strict diet. Besides normal water consumption, they drank five hundred milliliters of water half an hour before the three mandatory meals of the day. They continued this activity for eight consecutive weeks. The result of this little change in water consumption habits was outstanding. All the participants experienced decreased body weight, body mass index, and body fat. Other than that, they even stated appetite suppression. Many other studies also produced somewhat similar results.

The next benefit of drinking plain water is that it decreases a person's overall intake of liquid calories. The reason behind this is quite simple. Almost all of you know that water does not contain any calories. Accumulating liquid calories just by drinking juice, soda, sweetened tea, or coffee is quite easy. Thus if you fill up your glass with plain and natural water other than alternatives of higher calories like soda, juice, sweetened coffee, etc., then it can lower the chances of all over intake of calories in the liquid form. Many experts in this field state that you will intake a total number of two hundred and fifty fewer calories if you opt for water instead of a standard soft drink that is prepared by using a vending machine of twenty ounces. Another interesting fact is that diet soda does not contribute any calories. Now, if you replace such diet beverages and consume water, it would help in losing weight in some groups of individuals. Obese and overweight women who chose water by replacing diet beverages exhibited a huge reduction in weight.

Now, you may feel more excited after viewing the benefit of consuming plenty of water regularly. Water has the tendency to elevate calorie burning. A lot of trustworthy research has already been conducted for indicating the calorie-burning effect of water. In one study that took place in the year 2014, a total number of twelve individuals experienced an elevation in spending energy. The activity that they performed was drinking almost five hundred milliliters of room temperature and cold water. The percentage of calories burned by them was nearly two to three more than the usual rate. They burned the above-mentioned percentage of calories in the ninety minutes just after consuming the water. This essential, or you may say an integral element of all individual's lives, may also increase the total number of calories that are burned at the time of resting.

Another study that included overweight women showed positive results when they increased the quantity of water consumption to more than a liter each day. They continued this activity for a long period of twelve months, that is, one whole year. The result that they experienced or you may say enjoyed was an additional two kilograms of weight reduction. Various other similar and effective studies that monitored people who are overweight exhibited a decrease in BMI or body mass index, body weight, body fat, and waist circumference. The results turn out to be more impressive if the consumed water is cold. Thus, by now, you might have comprehended this simple yet effective fact that drinking a bit of cold water, not chilled, may enhance the calorie-burning effect of water to a great extent. It is because your body spends calories or energy by warming up the water that is necessary for digestion.

Your body will not be able to metabolize carbohydrates or stored fat without the help of water. Thus, water is highly necessary for burning fat. Lipolysis is the process that deals with metabolizing fat. Hydrolysis is known to be the first and foremost step of lipolysis. Hydrolysis occurs when the molecules of water interact with fats (triglycerides) for creating fatty acids and glycerol. A mini-study in the year 2016 found out that increasing the quantity of water consumption may result in enhanced lipolysis as well as fat loss. So, you need to drink an adequate quantity of water as it is essential not only for burning stored fat but also for fat from drink and food.

The quantity of water required by a person is dependent on various factors. Those factors include age, daily activity level, body temperature, body size, sun exposure, humidity level, health status, etc. The daily water consumption rate recommended by NAM or the National Academy of Medicine in the US is 3,700 milliliters of water for adult men and 2,700 milliliters for adult women. A lot of people feel worried when they think about including more water than the usual quantity. Are you also in the same group? Are you thinking about how you will escalate your water consumption capacity? Here are certain tips that might assist you in increasing your water intake.

- You may carry water while you move outside. Use any reusable bottle for this matter. Sip water while conversing with your colleagues or in between official meetings. Keep hydrating your body as much as possible.
- You may consume meals that are rich in a liquid, such as stews, unsweetened smoothies, curries as well as various types of soups. Try out different types of soups to break the monotonous taste. Think of tortilla

soup, minestrone, Chinese wonton, etc. When the soup is consumed before a meal, it assists in slowing down the pace of eating as well as curbs the appetite. You must not go for creamy soups as they are high in calories and fat.

- You may consume a glass full of water (eight ounces) after every meal. By doing so, you will have an idea of the quantity of water consumed throughout the day. So, maintain a measured glass.

- On days when the weather is too humid, warm, or sunny, drink an extra quantity of water.

- You may also keep a bottle filled with water and one glass near your bed so that you can drink water whenever you feel thirsty in between your resting time or while watching movies, web series, etc.

- While purchasing vegetables and fruits, you need to keep one thing in mind. Practice buying those veggies and fruits that have a high content of water. So, you may choose items such as grapes, different types of berries, tomatoes, melons, cucumbers, lettuce, celery, and a lot more.

So, drink, drink and keep drinking as much water as possible and enjoy a reduced body weight. Instead of following any popular diet to lose weight, simply make it a habit of drinking plenty of water.

Get Exposed to the Sun

A lot of you might think that exposure to the sun does not have any relation to weight loss. But you might be shocked to know that if you include this particular morning habit in your routine, the result will be appreciated. You need to open the curtains so that sunlight can peep in through the windows. You may also make it a habit to sit in the sun or spend a few more minutes in your garden early in the morning. Besides attaining a fresh and positive feeling, this habit will also help kick start losing weight. A small yet reliable study stated that if you stay exposed to moderate sunlight level and that too at any time of the day, it will leave a fruitful impact on your weight. Staying exposed to sunlight helps or rather is one of the best methods of meeting the requirements of vitamin D.

Studies have also been done related to this matter. It has been concluded that if a person receives the required quantity of vitamin D regularly, it may help in loss of weight as well as prevent regaining of the lost weight. A total number of 218 obese and overweight women were asked to participate in one such study. Those participants either took a placebo or vitamin D supplements for a year. When the study was terminated, the result was such that women who were able to meet the requirement of vitamin D lost nearly seven pounds or 3.2 kilograms of more weight on average than those whose vitamin D levels were inadequate.

Now, the fact that might strike your mind is what is the exact amount of staying exposed to sunlight. Well, it all depends on the season, the type of skin that you possess, your location, your daily activities, and a lot more. However, if you make it a habit of sitting outside your home in direct sunlight for nearly ten to fifteen minutes or allowing some sunlight to enter your room every morning, it will leave a beneficial impact on your weight loss.

Eat Foods That Consist of Fiber

Consuming food items that are rich in fiber may result in escalating satiety, that is, helps a person in feeling fuller and that too for a very long time. A particular kind of fiber, better known as viscous fiber, helps to suppress the appetite and is thus effective in losing extra weight. Viscous fiber decreases the intake of food as it boosts fullness. If the fiber is more viscous, then it shows better results in decreasing the usual appetite. When soluble viscous fibers like beta-glucans, guar gum, glucomannan, psyllium, pectin, etc., get connected with water, a gel is formed. Now, this specific gel helps develop the time required for absorbing nutrients as well as reduces the time for letting your stomach go empty. Thus, consuming more fiber may assist you in losing weight, even if other changes are not made in your regular meals. Viscous fiber is found only in different types of plant foods.

Here is a list of a few foods that are obtained from plants and are known to contain fiber.

- Brussels sprouts
- Green beans and lima beans
- Apples
- Asparagus
- Flax seeds
- Oranges
- Berries such as strawberries, raspberries, blackberries, etc.
- Sweet potatoes
- Chickpeas
- Pumpkin
- Squash
- Split peas
- Broccoli
- Guava
- Figs
- Pomegranate seeds
- Barley
- Banana
- Kiwi
- Pears

- Pureed avocados
- Lentils

This is a type of never-ending list as plant foods containing fiber go on and on. This little change in your regular meal has some other benefits other than aiding in weight loss. Intake of such foods regularly is also known to prevent constipation which is a major problem in the life of a huge number of people.

Serve Food Items on Smaller Plates

Using plates that are small in size may assist you in eating less amount of food. Serving foods on smaller plates makes the portion appear larger than usual. Whereas, if you use a larger plate, it will make your portion appear smaller, and that will insist you in adding more food to your plate. So, remove the larger plates from your kitchen and start using smaller ones. This is part of mindful eating, which we will discuss further in the next chapter.

Though this tiny habit may seem useless to some of you, you will get to see the positive result if you try it once. You may also try out one more habit related to plates. Serve healthy food items on larger plates and the ones that are less healthy on the smaller ones. Plates that are small in size may trick the brain and force it to think that you are consuming more food than the actual quantity. If you start eating unhealthy food items from comparatively smaller plates, you will eat less. Thus, choosing the size of plates for different foods is a great strategy for losing weight.

Chew the Food Thoroughly

First of all, you need to realize that your brain requires a little bit of time for processing that you have consumed enough food. To send that signal to your brain, you must utilize the habit of chewing the food thoroughly. If you practice thorough chewing, then you will eat at a slower pace than usual. This, in turn, will help you in decreasing the quantity of food intake, enhance the feeling of fullness, and include small portion sizes. The more quickly you complete your meal, it will affect your body weight.

As per the observations of a total number of twenty-three recent studies, people who are fast eaters and do not chew their food thoroughly tend to gain more weight than those who are slow eaters. Fast eaters also tend to become obese in future times.

Thus, a few effective and simple changes in your daily habits may prove to have an intense impact on weight loss, even if you do not follow any diet or strict calorie restriction. Start experimenting and enjoy weight loss!

Chapter 5: Your Guide to Mindful Eating

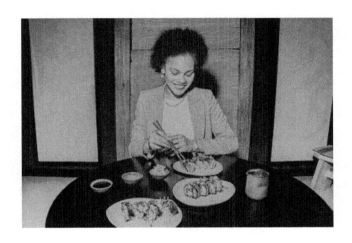

When you want to lose weight and become healthy, the most common thing or technique that people opt for is cutting down on what they eat. They go for dieting, which, we have already established, is not really a good thing to do because, in most cases, it turns out to be unhealthy for the person concerned. That is the reason the best option when you want to reduce weight is to practice mindful eating. You might or might not be familiar with this term, so let us talk about it in detail here. This chapter will try to answer all your pertinent questions regarding mindful eating and how it will help you in your weight loss journey. This chapter will also tell you what things that you should and should not do in order for you to get the best results from this practice. Let us then get into it in detail.

So, mindful eating is nothing but the technique that will help you be in control of everything that you eat and will ensure what your eating habits are. It helps you develop and practice healthy eating habits that do not harm your body and, in turn, helps you remain healthy and immune from diseases. Mindful eating also takes care of your mental health and sees to it that you are healthy both physically and emotionally. The entire idea of mindful eating has its roots in a Buddhist concept of mindfulness. To understand how you can practice mindful eating, first, let me briefly take you through what mindfulness is.

Mindfulness is a kind of meditating technique that ensures that you are capable of recognizing and coping with all your physical and emotional sensations and occurrences. Mindfulness is used to treat a lot of conditions in people, which includes depression, various kinds of eating disorders, other psychological problems like anxiety, and, at the same time, various kinds of food-related behavioral abnormalities. Mindful eating, then, is just a way that helps you own your eating experiences so that you can reach a state of complete attention when you are eating and so that you are fully aware of everything that your body is consuming.

Mindful eating will also let you experience all that you are feeling in their totality, like any cravings that you might be having, any physical cues that your body is sending you when you are eating, etc. This will help you to understand yourself better and what your body wants when you are eating or when you are thinking of consuming something. When you practice mindful eating, you help your body to replace all the automatic reactions and thoughts with more responsible and conscious ones and helps your body to get healthier and much better responses.

Why is Mindful Eating Necessary For You?

You might ask why it is at all essential for you to practice mindful eating. Well, the times that we live in are extremely busy and hectic. We do not get time to do one thing at a time and have to multitask most of the time to fit everything into our schedule. Similarly, the act of eating too has stopped being a mindful act and has been replaced with a mindless activity that many of us club with watching television or working on our computers. It is a common habit to make eating just an act that is associated with other things that we think are more important at that point. Also, we are given more than enough options of food items these days than what was available a few years ago. So many of us do not even give a thought to what we want to eat in actuality and take the first option that is available to us. Even thinking about sorting out from all the multiple options that we have can seem to be a task, so less and less time is spent on planning a proper meal or choosing something that we actually want.

When you do not spend enough time considering what you are eating and want to finish eating as soon as possible, that might lead to a lot of problems. It might make you binge eat, which is an act of mindlessly eating a lot and not even realizing it because you were not paying attention to what you are eating in the first place. You might understand much later that you have overeaten, and it will be already done by then. This is extremely harmful to your body. At the same time, when you do not pay much attention to the act of eating, you can also end up spending all your time on your work and not eating enough that your body needs to function properly.

That is precisely the reason you need to put your mind to eating and not make it a mere activity that can be dealt with lightly. When you put your mind on what you are eating, it becomes a conscious act, and all your effort goes on making sure you carry it out properly. Your senses become more alert, your body functions improve like your body's metabolism and also your digestive functions. You become able to differentiate between your actual hunger pangs and your non-hunger triggers. You get more used to your physical hunger cues and act upon them properly. When you start to understand what your hunger and non-hunger triggers are, you naturally become more equipped to handle all kinds of situations. As you take time to eat, you put all your senses at work in order for you to enjoy your food, and as a result, you can properly analyze how your food makes you feel and what effect it has on you. Apart from this, you become more equipped to handle the anxiety and guilt that can come when a person eats things that they were not planning to or were not supposed to eat.

Mindful eating helps you to be more in control of what you eat and what you don't. It helps you to take it into your own hands as to how you can lose weight. When you are not in control, you might have to rely on other people and factors regarding your weight loss journey. But when you practice mindful eating, you and no one else will have complete control, and that itself is the greatest thing of all. It is you who will be able to choose what you eat and how you respond to it. Your voluntary response is very crucial to your weight loss journey, and the faster you understand that, the better for you.

How is Weight Loss Connected to Mindful Eating?

In case you already do not know this, most people who start following a strict weight loss schedule or go on a very strict diet are not able to continue it in the long run, and they end up going back to that initial weight they started from. There are a lot of reasons for this. When you put your body through a very strict weight loss schedule like extreme dieting, for example, your body and your mind go through a lot. When you stop eating things that you like a lot, your body can experience a lot of cravings that might be really hard to ignore at times. As a result, many people can fall prey to things like emotional eating, where they eat something not because they are hungry but because they haven't had that food item for a long time.

They can also fall prey to binge eating, where they do not put any thought into what they are eating or how much they are eating, but they do so mindlessly. Some people even fail to understand non-hunger food triggers and give in to that. As a result, there comes a lot of anxiety and guilt when that happens. When all of these above-mentioned things happen, weight gain is a very common thing. Even if you had managed to lose a lot of weight initially, you could gain that weight over a short period of time because you are not mindful of what you are eating.

Mindful eating, as I have already mentioned, is related to the practice of mindfulness which helps you own your actions and be in control. The reason I am telling this is that when you are not mindful, you can undergo a lot of stress and that itself can be a reason as to why you are gaining weight. Reducing stress is essential when you want to lose weight, and that can be done when you practice mindfulness and practice mindful eating.

What Should You Do in Order to Practice Mindful Eating?

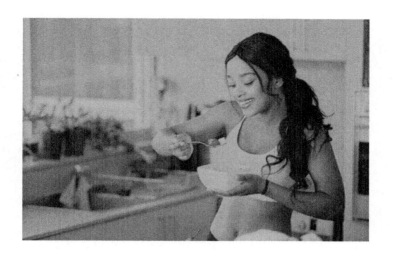

Now that we have discussed certain aspects of mindful eating and why it is so important for you, let me take you through some of the ways in which you can practice mindful eating in real life and be benefitted from the results, one of which is losing weight.

Do Not Rush With Your Food

One of the best ways to practice mindful eating is to put all your concentration on what you are eating and to not rush with your food. Many of us might have the habit of eating in a hurry and not even noticing properly what we are eating. Maybe once in a while, when you go out to eat with someone, or it is a special occasion, that you actually have some time in your hands while eating, and then you take notice. But other than that, most of the time, when you eat, you eat in a rush. Given that all of us lead a very busy life, many might have the habit of giving the least amount of time to eat. Getting up late, preparing for work, and then hurriedly gulping down some juice or heading out with a piece of bread to have on the go is not really a very uncommon sight. People do it all the time. This is something that you need to stop doing immediately.

If you think that you aren't getting enough time in the morning, maybe consider getting up a bit early so that you do not have to skip breakfast. During lunch at work, take that time off because you are supposed to and eat a proper meal. Do not rush with your food, always giving the excuse of "not having enough time" always. When you do not put enough thoughts into what you are eating, you tend to gain weight. When your mind is somewhere else, and you are not giving enough time to chew your food properly, it does not get digested well. Your metabolism will get messed up this way. Rushing through your meal makes your mind and body confused, and as a result, you can gain weight due to the food not getting digested properly. You might also experience things like indigestion in case you eat too fast without chewing it properly. You have gastritis when you skip your meals and much more. That is the reason, when you want to practice mindfulness, do not rush with your food. Instead, take some time to properly see and chew what you are eating.

Avoid All Kinds of Distraction When You Are Eating

I cannot ever put enough stress on this subject, and that is, you simply cannot entertain any kind of distractions when you are eating. Many of us might have the habit of watching television or working at the side when we are eating. This is a very problematic habit. Your body might have to go through a lot of problems when you do that. You see, you have a brain to think about all your stuff, and it takes decisions regarding the functioning of your body. Your body needs the correct directions from your brain to do a certain work thoroughly. It is not possible for your body to see to it that everything is being done properly like the way they are supposed to when your brain is so confused. When you are watching television, your brain wants to concentrate on that and enjoy whatever you are watching. When you are working, your brain, quite similarly, wants to concentrate on that and it gets really confused when you try to push other things on their way.

When you are eating, your brain needs to understand that that is what you are concentrating on, and only then will it be able to let your body's metabolism work properly and help your body to get all the nutrients properly and digest your food properly. When your mind is in two places or over multiple things, it just makes it all the more difficult for your body to do any of those work properly. Not only are there chances of making mistakes in your work, but you can also gain a lot of weight that way simply because your body will not digest the food properly. So make sure you do only one thing at a time. If you are eating, make sure you are doing only that so that you can digest everything properly.

Listen to All the Physical Hunger Cues

Your body has its own way of telling you that it is hungry, and that is an important thing that you most definitely should not avoid. You might be really busy with a lot of things, but your body knows when it needs food and when you avoid that, it has its own ways to let you know that. It might differ from person to person. Some might feel a pain or a kind of discomfort in their bellies which tells them that it has been a long time since they last ate, and it is time now that they should eat their next meal. For others, it might be something else. But no matter what that sign or cue is that your body is giving you, you should not avoid it. You see, your body has its own way of staying fit. You might feel that skipping a meal is alright because you will eat later. But that is not the ideal way your body works. That is not the way your body can stay healthy.

You might feel that eating later is a proper option because you have habituated yourself to ignore these physical cues and tolerate any discomfort that you might be feeling at that point. But what happens because of this is really not ideal and very harmful for your body. Your body needs fat to get the energy to spend the entire day properly. Now, when it does not get the proper amount of food at the proper time, it thinks that the less irregular food that it is getting is all the food that it will get. So what it tries to do is store that as fat in your body for it to get the energy it needs. As a result of this, you tend to get fat when you do not eat at regular intervals and make your body wait for longer periods of time to get a proper meal. So, when your body gives you physical cues that it is hungry, take a short break from what you were doing and eat. Let your body get all the nutrients that it needs and not convert everything into fat. That way you will be healthy and be able to maintain your weight as well.

Stop Eating Once You Are Full

Just like your body will tell you when it is hungry, it will also tell you when it is full. That is also an important thing to notice and act accordingly. No matter how much you like eating that particular food item, your body has a limit to how much it can take in, and you have to stop at that. Your body is not a neverending void where an endless amount of food can go and possibly disappear. There is a limit to how much food is healthy for you to eat. Beyond that, it is unhealthy for you. Your body will start showing internal and external signs of discomfort and, in most cases, medical signs like indigestion, obesity, and in worse cases, high blood sugar or even high cholesterol levels when you do not eat what is healthy for your body and eat more than what you are supposed to.

When you eat even after you are full, there arises a lot of problems in your body that you should not have to deal with if you can just remember to not overeat. It might so be that you really like what you are eating. In that case, instead of eating everything all at once, keep the rest of the portion for later and stop when you see that your body is full. Give your body the time it needs to properly digest what you eat. You will gain a lot of weight if you do not stop overeating. An average human body takes about three to four hours to fully digest a proper meal that you consume. You need to give yourself that time. Only then will your body be able to fully take in all the nutrients without making you obese. Neither should you force yourself or let anyone else force you to eat once you are full. When you start doing that, that is, eating only till you are full, you will see how easily your metabolism will improve and how easily you will be able to maintain your weight without falling ill.

Differentiate Between Actual Hunger And Non-Hunger Triggers

It is possible for you to have a lot of non-hunger triggers, but you should be able to understand them from the real ones and not act upon them. You should only act upon your actual hunger triggers as otherwise, you can gain a lot of weight. Non-hunger triggers can be of various kinds. You might want to eat something because your friend is eating them or because you wanted to have that for some time, but just because you were not getting it, you go for it even though you are not hungry at all. You might eat something now, thinking you have a long day ahead and you will not get time to eat a proper meal for the entire day. You might eat something even though you are not hungry just because it looks so good and it is too hard to resist it. You might eat something because that is your comfort food, and when you are anxious, you think that will help you to calm down. There could be a thousand possible reasons and triggers for you to indulge in food even when you are not hungry.

But you have to understand what is good for you and what is not. Indulge only those triggers that come from actual hunger. Eat only when you are hungry, and your body actually needs the food, not when you simply want to have it no matter how full you are. Do not push extra food in your belly as not only is that bad for your health, but it will also lead to a lot of weight gain. So next time, when you feel like eating something, ask yourself whether you are actually hungry or not. If the answer is yes, then you can consider having it. But if the answer is no, then either skip it completely or if you want, keep it for later so that when you are actually hungry, you can have it then. This will also help your body digest it easily, and it will not have a negative impact on your health or weight.

Engage All Your Senses While Eating

When you are having a meal, make sure that you are engaging all your senses in it. That is, see properly what you are eating. Do not go about eating anything just because you have to. See properly. Take in the smell of what you are having. Unless you do that, how will you know whether you like it or not? It is important because unless you like the smell, the taste will automatically go down on your measurement scale than what it would have been if you had liked the smell of it. After that, when you taste your food, do not go about gulping it down. Chew it properly and try to see what you think of the texture of what you are eating and what you think of all the flavors in it. You have to take into account that because otherwise, there is no point even eating anything that has been cooked with care. If you are to not do any of these, you could have just eaten plain boiled vegetables and be done with it.

You might think, what is the point of all this when your aim is to lose weight. Well, your aim might be to lose weight, but the food that you are consuming has a lot of purposes. It is going in your body and providing you with nourishment. At the same time, when you have those food items that you like, it gives you a lot of emotional satisfaction. That is where the entire concept of comfort food is based. People resort to food at times when they feel low or anxious or when they want to relax. Every person has a specific kind of food that they like a lot and consuming that gives them genuine happiness. That is the reason you have to engage all your senses when you are eating. Be in control of what you are eating and when you are eating that. Let that be a meaningful experience and not something that you are forcefully doing. When you are happy with the food that you just had, when those flavors make you feel good emotionally, it will have a positive impact on your physical health as well. Your body will be more receptive towards digesting it when it is aware of what you are having.

Learn to Deal With the Guilt And the Anxiety About Eating

This is one of the essential elements of mindful eating. It is absolutely normal and also very common to eat things once in a while that you are not supposed to. Maybe you could not control yourself and had a pastry or a bar of chocolate when you had promised yourself that you would not do that for a month. Maybe you were feeling really low, and you had a pizza as that gives you comfort. While you were doing it, you did not feel bad. Instead, you wanted that comfort, and as you were craving that food, you were really happy while eating it. But after you have finished eating it, now your brain is giving you mixed signals. You start feeling guilty that you did something you were not supposed to. Probably you were very serious about your diet, maybe you still are, and the fact that you broke that rule and consumed something which made a lot of earlier effort to lose weight go to waste is what is making you feel frustrated with yourself, and you are feeling guilty now. This guilt will slowly start making you feel anxious, and all over, it will start having a negative effect on you.

This is something that you need to stop doing. As I have mentioned earlier, this is completely normal, and it can happen to anyone. We are all human beings, and going out of the way once in a while is absolutely fine. Tell yourself that you are in control of what you are eating. When you are able to successfully maintain a certain food habit for so long, you will also be able to do it again. If you are too strict with yourself, that will just make you feel like opting out. What you can do instead is make yourself a flexible routine where you allow yourself to have things that your body craves occasionally. When your body knows that it will not be deprived of things that it likes, it will not have the tendency to want it all the time. When you feel anxious, your brain and your body start feeling that they have done something really wrong and impact your health negatively. It can also happen that in that state of anxiousness, you start eating those food items more than you would have done otherwise, and this cycle of eating and feeling guilty and eating more will continue. Instead, give yourself a break once in a while and eat everything in moderation so that all your cravings are satisfied and you do not need to feel bad about eating anything.

Try to Maintain Your Overall Health And Well Being

The idea behind eating is not only to satisfy your hunger. It is to see that what you are consuming is helping you to maintain a healthy mind as well. You need to feel good about yourself, and you need to look after your well-being. You have to constantly remind yourself that it is you who controls what you eat and not the other way round. Do not go about eating things that are not good for your health. Certain things do not suit some people. If that is the case for you, then you should avoid them at all costs and not make your body go through unnecessary problems. You are more than intelligent to know what is good for you and what is not. Your well-being is not only restricted to what you eat in the form of food items but also other things that you consume, like alcohol or nicotine if you smoke. These are things that are not good for your health, be it physical and mental health, and that is the reason you need to keep a check on everything that you are consuming as a whole.

Your goal should be to consume things that improve your overall well-being and helps you to lead a healthy life. You cannot jeopardize that at any cost. Do not say yes to go for another round of drinks if you know that will make you fall ill just because your friends are telling you to. Do not indulge in smoking if that makes you feel uneasy just because everyone else around you does that. What others are doing is their priority, and how they want to maintain their health is also their lookout. What you should be concerned with is how you are dealing with maintaining a healthy body and a healthy life. Weight loss might be your primary aim, but it cannot be at the cost of you giving up on other things. Your body needs to be strong and not only be of a certain amount of weight. Your body needs to have strong immunity, and you need to be healthy before anything else. That is the reason, even when you are trying to lose weight, do not opt for techniques that hamper your health or makes you drastically lose out on calories while destroying your immune system and causing other problems.

Analyze What You Are Feeling And What Effects Food Has on You

Mindful eating is about many things, and one of them is about you truly feeling what impact food has on you. When you make eating an act of complete experience for yourself, you will get much more than mere sustenance from it. Ask yourself what it is that you feel when you eat something that you like. What does it make you feel? For some people, it can only be about satisfying their hunger. For some, it might be an act of habit. For some, it can be an occasion of getting immersed in taste and smell. For some, it could be another instance of losing control and then later feeling guilty about it. For some, it can be something else as well. It is completely a subjective matter as to what food makes you feel and what effect eating has on you. But no matter what effect it has on you, what is important is that you do not ignore that. Be it good or bad, it is necessary that you take notice of that and try and analyze it in detail.

It is important that you know how your body reacts to food. If you see that certain kinds of food items are not making you feel good, ask yourself why that is so. Remember that if your body is rejecting any food and you force it on yourself, it can have a lot of negative impacts on your health. Similarly, when you see that certain kinds of food make you feel good, try and understand why that is so. If that is making you feel good, quite naturally, it will have a positive impact on your body and on your mind. It is very helpful that you know your preference and creates your own palate. Your taste and preferences are solely your decision, and no one should force you to consume things that you do not want or keep you away from things that you like. So when you analyze what effect food has on you and find out what it makes you feel, your body is more at ease, and it helps you in the weight loss process as well.

Appreciate What You Are Eating

You can never expect to lose weight unless you appreciate the things that you are eating. Consuming food is as much a physical thing as it is a psychological thing. You need to be grateful for the food that you are having, and you need to be genuinely appreciative of the fact that you have food on your plate. How your body physically functions has got to do a lot with how it feels emotionally. When you are not appreciative of things, food that you eat in this case, your body will not accept it well. But when you are genuinely appreciative of what you are eating, your mind knows that it means something important to you, and then your body, too, will react to it in a positive way. Even if you are eating things that you like, losing weight will not be a problem because your mind will know what you want, and your body will react in a cooperative manner.

The ultimate goal in life should be to lead a healthy life, one that is free of illness and problems. Well, certain external things are not in our control. But what is in our control is the food that we consume. So, when we can eat things that will add to our well-being and health, only a fool will reject it. What is then the most sensible thing to do is, to be honest with yourself and appreciate what you have on your plate. Even if you want to lose weight, you won't be able to do it unless you know the value of what you already have. So when you want to practice mindful eating, learn to appreciate what you are eating before you do anything else.

Things That Mindful Eating Helps You With

Apart from helping you to lose weight, mindful eating has been proved to reduce other things as well, and those are –

External Eating	An act of external eating is when you eat not because you are hungry but because of responding to environmental factors and other food-related cues. For example, the smell or the sight of food makes you drawn towards it, and it becomes difficult for you to resist eating it.

	With mindful eating, you will be able to reason out with yourself and not give in to these external triggers.
Emotional Eating	We all are aware that food is a great way to relieve yourself of stress. Also, it is one of the most common ways in which people celebrate something good. So, be it a happy situation or a sad one, or when you feel anxious, or you are in need of comfort, you might resort to food. This is not a healthy thing as eating even when you are not hungry but due to some

	psychological factor is never good for the body. Mindful eating helps you reason out with that as well and remain in control.
Binge Eating	Mindful eating helps you to stop this habit of binge eating as well. When you are too busy with other work, and you cannot give a lot of thought to what you are eating, you can tend to binge eat, and that leads to weight gain. You need to stop doing it and put your mind on what you are eating.

I hope this has helped to clear some of your doubts regarding mindful eating. Of course, there is a lot more to it than this, but this is enough information for you to get a clear idea about what mindful eating is and how it can help you lose weight. The main factor then is to be conscious at all times regarding what you are eating and to be in control of your food habits. It will then become easy for you to not only lose weight and get to the proper shape but remain healthy and maintain a fit body. I hope you can greatly benefit from this, and when you start to practice mindful eating, I hope you will be able to get to the weight you desire for yourself.

Conclusion

Thank you for making it through to the end of *Stop Dieting, Change Your Life and Lose Weight*. Let's hope it was informative and able to provide you with all of the tools you need to achieve your goals, whatever they may be.

Let me first congratulate you on reaching the end of this book. It is a very courageous thing that you have done by making the decision of embarking on this journey of losing weight through healthy habits. There are many people around us that want to lose weight, but not everyone has the courage to get up and actually change things for the better. So, today, I wish you all the best for your future, and I really hope you keep up the habits you learned in this book.

This choice that you have made to lead a better life will also enable you to remain in a balanced state of mind. I hope this book has been successful in teaching you the right way to lose weight and also opened your eyes to how diets can be harmful. Always remember that if you want to change something, it is you who has to make that decision and take some action. No one else can do it for you. This is your time and, above all, your life.

Finally, if you found this book useful in any way, a review on Amazon is always appreciated!